UNLOCK YOUR BODY'S TRUE POTENTIAL

Stronger, Longer

The Anti-Aging Power of Strength Training & The Hormone Code

QAYYUM NEVREKAR

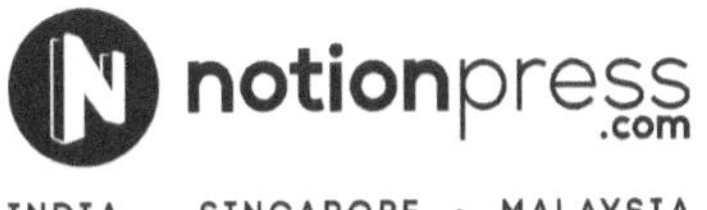

Chapter 1: Strength Training and Hormonal Health for Longevity

Aging brings muscle loss, weaker bones, and hormonal shifts that affect energy and metabolism. Strength training, paired with hormone balance, plays a key role in staying strong, preventing disease, and maintaining vitality. This book provides an easy-to-follow guide for Indians to incorporate resistance training and hormone optimization into daily life for long-term health.

Key Focus Areas

- ➤ How strength training supports longevity and muscle retention.

- ➤ The role of hormones in fitness and aging.

- ➤ Practical training and dietary strategies for Indians.

- ➤ A sustainable fitness plan for lifelong health.

Chapter 2: Bone Health & Injury Prevention

- ➤ Strength training's role in preventing osteoporosis and fractures.

- ➤ Best exercises for increasing bone density.

➤ How to modify workouts for joint issues and recovery.

Chapter 3: Hormones & Strength Training

➤ How testosterone, growth hormone, and insulin influence muscle growth.

➤ The negative impact of high cortisol on fat gain.

➤ The connection between insulin resistance and energy levels.

Chapter 4: Boosting Testosterone Naturally

➤ The importance of strength training for testosterone levels.

➤ Indian dietary habits that enhance testosterone production.

➤ The role of sleep and stress reduction.

Chapter 5: Managing Cortisol & Stress

➤ How chronic stress disrupts muscle growth and fat metabolism.

➤ The benefits of yoga, meditation, and sleep.

➤ Exercise modifications to prevent overtraining and burnout.

Chapter 6: Balancing Estrogen & Testosterone

- ➤ Understanding estrogen dominance in men and women.

- ➤ The impact of estrogen on fat distribution.

- ➤ Natural ways to maintain hormone balance.

Chapter 7: Strength Training & Insulin Sensitivity

- ➤ How lifting weights improves glucose metabolism.

- ➤ Exercise and dietary strategies to prevent diabetes.

- ➤ The benefits of intermittent fasting for hormonal health.

Chapter 8: Thyroid Health & Energy Regulation

- ➤ The thyroid's role in metabolism and fat loss.

- ➤ How strength training supports thyroid function.

- ➤ Nutritional guidelines for maintaining a healthy thyroid.

Chapter 9: Creating an Effective Training Plan

- ➤ Key resistance exercises for aging adults.

> ➤ How to progress in strength training safely.

> ➤ Adjusting workouts based on age and experience.

Chapter 10: Nutrition for Strength & Hormonal Balance

> ➤ Best protein sources in an Indian diet.

> ➤ The role of micronutrients in muscle recovery.

> ➤ How traditional Indian diets can be optimized for longevity.

Chapter 11: Debunking Strength Training Myths

> ➤ Strength training is not just for bodybuilders.

> ➤ Lifting heavy weights does not make women bulky.

> ➤ Older adults can safely engage in resistance training.

Chapter 12: Supplements & Natural Adaptogens

> ➤ Indian herbs like Ashwagandha and Shatavari for hormone support.

> ➤ Best supplements for muscle growth and recovery.

> How to use supplements safely and effectively.

Chapter 13: Recovery & Regeneration

> Why rest and recovery are as important as training.

> The benefits of massage, stretching, and active recovery.

> How sleep influences hormone balance and muscle repair.

Chapter 14: Strength Training & Hormonal Health in India

> The impact of Indian dietary habits and cultural perceptions.

> Overcoming lifestyle challenges to build strength.

> Making fitness a long-term priority in Indian households.

Chapter 15: Long-Term Strength & Wellness Strategy

> Staying consistent with workouts as you age.

> How to track progress and make adjustments.

> ➤ Developing a sustainable fitness mindset for lifelong health.

Conclusion: The Path to Strength & Longevity

> ➤ Key takeaways on strength training and hormone optimization.

> ➤ The importance of patience and long-term commitment.

> ➤ A practical roadmap to aging strong and staying fit.

CHAPTER 1

STRENGTH TRAINING AND HORMONAL HEALTH FOR LONGEVITY

Aging brings muscle loss, weaker bones, and hormonal shifts that affect energy and metabolism. Strength training, paired with hormone balance, plays a key role in staying strong, preventing disease, and maintaining vitality. This book provides an easy-to-follow guide for Indians to incorporate resistance training and hormone optimization into daily life for long-term health.

Key Focus Areas

How Strength Training Supports Longevity and Muscle Retention

Strength training is crucial in maintaining muscle mass as we age. Without resistance training, muscle atrophy (sarcopenia) begins as early as the 30s, leading to decreased strength, mobility issues, and increased risk of falls and fractures. Progressive resistance training helps to:

> ➢ Preserve lean muscle mass and prevent age-related muscle loss.

> ➢ Enhance mobility, flexibility, and posture.

> ➢ Improve metabolism, keeping body fat in check while increasing energy levels.

> ➢ Strengthen tendons, ligaments, and bones, reducing the risk of osteoporosis and joint degeneration.

> ➢ Promote independence and better quality of life in later years.

For Indians, integrating strength training into daily routines can be achieved through traditional bodyweight exercises, yoga, and gym-based resistance training. Even **30 minutes of strength training, 3-4 times a week**, can significantly improve muscle retention and strength over time.

The Role of Hormones in Fitness and Aging

Hormones act as the body's natural regulators for muscle growth, fat metabolism, and overall energy levels. As people age, hormonal imbalances contribute to muscle loss, weight gain, and sluggishness. Some key hormones affected by aging include:

- **Testosterone:** Declines with age, leading to muscle loss and reduced recovery.

- **Growth Hormone:** Helps with muscle repair and fat metabolism but diminishes over time.

- **Cortisol:** Chronic stress increases cortisol levels, causing muscle breakdown and fat accumulation.

- **Estrogen:** Plays a role in fat distribution and bone health, particularly for women.

- **Insulin:** Affects how the body utilizes energy, with poor insulin sensitivity leading to fat storage and metabolic diseases.

By implementing strength training and dietary changes, Indians can naturally regulate these hormones to enhance fitness and longevity.

Practical Training and Dietary Strategies for Indians

Indians face unique dietary and lifestyle challenges, from carbohydrate-heavy diets to limited protein intake. To optimize strength and hormonal balance:

Training Strategies

- ➢ **Compound Movements:** Squats, deadlifts, lunges, and push-ups to engage multiple muscle groups.

- ➢ **Progressive Overload:** Gradually increasing weight or resistance to improve strength.

- ➢ **Functional Training:** Exercises mimicking daily activities to enhance mobility and prevent injuries.

- ➢ **Recovery and Stretching:** Yoga and flexibility exercises to reduce stiffness and promote longevity.

Dietary Strategies

- ➢ **Protein-Rich Diet:** Lean meats, dairy, eggs, legumes, and plant-based proteins to support muscle growth.

- ➢ **Healthy Fats:** Ghee, coconut oil, nuts, and seeds for hormonal balance.

- ➢ **Complex Carbohydrates:** Whole grains, millets, and fibrous vegetables for sustained energy.

> **Micronutrients:** Zinc, magnesium, and vitamin D to support bone health and hormonal function.

A well-structured Indian diet, focusing on **whole foods and protein-rich meals**, combined with resistance training, ensures optimal fitness outcomes.

A Sustainable Fitness Plan for Lifelong Health

Sustainability is key in maintaining fitness and hormonal balance long-term. A structured approach to training and diet includes:

> **Setting Realistic Goals:** Focus on consistency rather than drastic changes.

> **Building Habits:** Incorporating physical activity into daily routines, such as using stairs, stretching, or short workouts.

> **Tracking Progress:** Keeping a journal or using fitness apps to monitor improvements.

> **Adapting Workouts to Age:** Adjusting intensity based on individual needs and energy levels.

> ➢ **Mind-Body Connection:** Using meditation, mindfulness, and stress reduction techniques to complement training.

By adopting a well-rounded strength training regimen and hormonal optimization strategies, Indians can age gracefully, remain strong, and lead a healthier life for years to come.

CHAPTER 2

BONE HEALTH & INJURY PREVENTION

Strength Training's Role in Preventing Osteoporosis and Fractures

As we age, bone density naturally declines, increasing the risk of fractures and osteoporosis. Strength training is one of the most effective ways to improve bone density and prevent injuries. Weight-bearing exercises stimulate osteoblasts (bone-building cells), leading to stronger bones.

Benefits of Strength Training for Bone Health

- Enhances bone mineral density, reducing fracture risk.

- Strengthens supporting muscles, reducing falls and injuries.

- Improves balance, coordination, and joint stability.

- Increases mobility and independence in older adults.

Best Exercises for Increasing Bone Density

Weight-Bearing Exercises

- **Squats:** Strengthen the lower body and enhance bone density in hips and legs.

- **Lunges:** Improve balance and strengthen the femur, reducing fracture risks.

- **Deadlifts:** Engage the posterior chain, improving overall strength and stability.

- **Overhead Press:** Strengthens the shoulders and spine, reducing the risk of vertebral fractures.

Bodyweight & Functional Movements

- **Push-ups:** Enhance upper-body strength and improve posture.

- **Step-ups:** Strengthen the legs and challenge balance.

- **Planks:** Build core strength, supporting overall stability.

- **Yoga Poses (e.g., Warrior Pose):** Improve flexibility and strengthen bones over time.

How to Modify Workouts for Joint Issues and Recovery

Aging individuals or those with joint pain should take a customized approach to training. High-impact movements can be modified for comfort and safety.

Low-Impact Strength Training Options

- **Resistance Bands:** Provide controlled resistance without joint strain.

- **Seated Strength Training:** Allows muscle activation while reducing joint pressure.

- **Aquatic Exercises:** Water buoyancy supports joints, allowing resistance training with minimal impact.

Recovery and Injury Prevention Techniques

- **Proper Warm-Up:** Dynamic stretches and mobility drills before workouts.

- **Adequate Rest:** Allowing recovery between workouts to avoid overuse injuries.

- **Foam Rolling & Massage:** Reduces stiffness and improves circulation.

> **Consuming Calcium & Vitamin D:** Supports bone remodeling and repair.

Bone Health and Strength Training in the Indian Context

Indians, particularly postmenopausal women and elderly individuals, are at a higher risk of osteoporosis due to genetic factors, dietary habits, and limited sun exposure.

Dietary Adjustments for Bone Health

> **Increase Calcium Intake:** Dairy, leafy greens, and fortified plant-based milk.

> **Enhance Vitamin D Levels:** Sun exposure and supplementation.

> **Consume Protein-Rich Foods:** Lentils, paneer, eggs, and lean meats to support muscle and bone health.

> **Reduce Processed Foods:** Minimize excessive salt, sugar, and carbonated drinks that deplete bone minerals.

By integrating strength training with proper nutrition and recovery techniques, Indians can maintain strong bones, prevent injuries, and ensure long-term health and mobility.

CHAPTER 3

HORMONES & STRENGTH TRAINING

How Testosterone, Growth Hormone, and Insulin Influence Muscle Growth

Hormones play a crucial role in muscle development, fat metabolism, and energy levels. Understanding how these hormones interact with strength training can help optimize muscle gain and overall fitness.

Testosterone: The Muscle-Building Hormone

- Testosterone is a key anabolic hormone responsible for muscle growth, recovery, and fat metabolism.

- It enhances protein synthesis, allowing muscles to repair and grow after resistance training.

- Declining testosterone levels with age can lead to muscle loss and fat gain.

How to Boost Testosterone Naturally

- ➤ Strength training with compound exercises like squats, deadlifts, and bench presses.

- ➤ Consuming healthy fats from nuts, seeds, and olive oil to support testosterone production.

- ➤ Prioritizing high-quality sleep, as most testosterone production occurs during deep sleep.

Growth Hormone: The Regenerator

- ➤ Growth hormone (GH) stimulates cell growth, muscle repair, and fat burning.

- ➤ GH levels peak during deep sleep and intense exercise, particularly high-intensity interval training (HIIT) and strength workouts.

Ways to Enhance Growth Hormone

- ➤ Engaging in heavy resistance training and HIIT workouts.

- ➤ Practicing intermittent fasting, which has been shown to increase GH production.

- ➤ Reducing sugar intake, as high insulin levels can suppress GH secretion.

Insulin: The Energy Regulator

> ➤ Insulin plays a dual role: it helps shuttle nutrients into cells for muscle growth but can also promote fat storage if not managed properly.

> ➤ Strength training enhances insulin sensitivity, allowing muscles to absorb glucose more efficiently and reducing the risk of diabetes.

Strategies to Optimize Insulin Sensitivity

> ➤ Performing resistance training at least three times a week.

> ➤ Prioritizing complex carbohydrates like brown rice, quinoa, and whole grains.

> ➤ Avoiding processed sugars and excessive snacking.

The Negative Impact of High Cortisol on Fat Gain

Cortisol, commonly known as the stress hormone, can have a significant impact on body composition. While short-term cortisol spikes help with energy production, chronic elevation can lead to muscle breakdown and fat storage.

Effects of High Cortisol

➤ Increases abdominal fat storage.

➤ Suppresses testosterone and growth hormone production.

➤ Breaks down muscle tissue, leading to reduced strength and performance.

Ways to Reduce Cortisol Levels

➤ Incorporating relaxation techniques like meditation, deep breathing, and yoga.

➤ Limiting excessive caffeine consumption, which can spike cortisol.

➤ Prioritizing quality sleep to regulate cortisol rhythms.

➤ Engaging in low-impact activities like walking and stretching to balance stress levels.

The Connection Between Insulin Resistance and Energy Levels

Insulin resistance occurs when the body's cells become less responsive to insulin, causing blood sugar levels to rise. This leads to:

- ➤ Increased fat storage, particularly in the abdominal area.

- ➤ Reduced energy levels and constant fatigue.

- ➤ Higher risk of metabolic disorders, including Type 2 diabetes.

How Strength Training Improves Insulin Sensitivity

- ➤ Resistance training helps muscles absorb glucose more effectively, reducing insulin resistance.

- ➤ HIIT workouts have been shown to improve glucose metabolism within weeks.

- ➤ Engaging in post-meal walks helps lower blood sugar levels naturally.

Dietary Changes for Insulin Sensitivity

- ➤ Increasing fiber intake through vegetables, legumes, and whole grains.

- ➤ Avoiding high-glycemic foods that cause blood sugar spikes.

> ➤ Consuming protein with meals to slow carbohydrate absorption and stabilize energy levels.

Final Takeaways: Balancing Hormones for Strength and Longevity

> ➤ Strength training not only builds muscle but also optimizes hormone function.

> ➤ Prioritizing testosterone, growth hormone, and insulin regulation enhances muscle gain and energy levels.

> ➤ Managing cortisol through stress reduction, sleep, and diet is essential for preventing fat gain.

> ➤ Improving insulin sensitivity through training and proper nutrition ensures sustained energy and metabolic health.

By implementing these hormone-focused strategies, individuals can achieve sustainable strength, better health, and longevity through strength training.

CHAPTER 4

BOOSTING TESTOSTERONE NATURALLY

The Importance of Strength Training for Testosterone Levels

Testosterone plays a crucial role in muscle growth, fat loss, energy production, and overall well-being. As men and women age, testosterone levels naturally decline, leading to decreased muscle mass, increased body fat, and lower energy levels. Strength training is one of the most effective natural ways to enhance testosterone levels.

How Strength Training Boosts Testosterone

> **Compound Movements:** Exercises like squats, deadlifts, and bench presses stimulate large muscle groups and increase testosterone production.

> **Progressive Overload:** Increasing resistance over time signals the body to produce more testosterone.

> **High-Intensity Workouts:** Short bursts of intense exercise (e.g., HIIT) have been shown to elevate testosterone levels more than long-duration cardio.

> **Training Volume & Frequency:** Training large muscle groups 3-4 times per week enhances hormone production.

Indian Dietary Habits That Enhance Testosterone Production

Diet plays a crucial role in testosterone levels. Indians often consume carbohydrate-heavy meals, which can affect insulin and testosterone balance. However, incorporating the right foods can support natural hormone production.

Testosterone-Boosting Foods in Indian Diet

> **Healthy Fats:** Ghee, coconut oil, almonds, and walnuts promote hormone synthesis.

> **Protein Sources:** Paneer, lentils, eggs, and lean meats support muscle growth and testosterone production.

> **Zinc & Magnesium-Rich Foods:** Pumpkin seeds, chickpeas, and spinach help in testosterone synthesis.

> **Vitamin D Sources:** Sun exposure, dairy, and fortified plant-based milk aid in testosterone regulation.

Foods That Lower Testosterone

> **Refined Carbs & Sugars:** Excess sugar and processed foods contribute to insulin resistance and lower testosterone.

> **Soy-Based Products:** Excessive soy consumption may lead to estrogen dominance.

> **Alcohol & Processed Foods:** Excessive alcohol disrupts hormone production and liver detoxification.

The Role of Sleep and Stress Reduction in Testosterone Production

Testosterone is primarily produced during deep sleep. Chronic stress and poor sleep habits can disrupt hormone production, leading to imbalances.

Optimizing Sleep for Higher Testosterone

> **Maintain a Regular Sleep Schedule:** Sleep for 7-9 hours every night to allow proper hormone release.

> ➤ **Create a Sleep-Inducing Environment:** Reduce blue light exposure, avoid caffeine before bed, and keep the room cool.

> ➤ **Supplement with Melatonin & Magnesium:** These help regulate sleep and support testosterone levels.

Managing Stress to Maintain Testosterone

> ➤ **Meditation & Yoga:** Practices like pranayama and mindfulness reduce cortisol levels, balancing testosterone production.

> ➤ **Regular Exercise:** Physical activity improves mood and lowers stress-related hormone fluctuations.

> ➤ **Adaptogenic Herbs:** Ashwagandha and Shilajit, commonly used in Ayurvedic medicine, help regulate stress hormones and enhance testosterone.

Testosterone Optimization Strategies for Indians

1. **Follow a Strength Training Routine:**

   o Train with compound movements at least three times per week.

- o Use moderate-to-heavy weights with 6-12 repetitions per set.

2. **Adopt a Nutrient-Dense Diet:**

   - o Include healthy fats, adequate protein, and micronutrient-rich foods.

   - o Reduce sugar and processed food intake.

3. **Prioritize Sleep and Recovery:**

   - o Maintain a consistent sleep routine.

   - o Avoid stressors and engage in relaxation techniques.

4. **Use Natural Testosterone Boosters:**

   - o Include Ayurvedic supplements like Ashwagandha, Shilajit, and Gokshura.

5. **Stay Active Beyond the Gym:**

   - o Engage in outdoor activities, walking, and sports to enhance overall hormone function.

Final Takeaways: Achieving Optimal Testosterone Levels Naturally

- ➤ Strength training is the most effective way to naturally enhance testosterone production.

> ➤ An Indian diet can be optimized for testosterone support by including healthy fats, proteins, and essential vitamins.

> ➤ Quality sleep and stress management play a critical role in maintaining hormone balance.

> ➤ Traditional Ayurvedic herbs can be beneficial in supporting testosterone levels.

By integrating these strategies into daily life, individuals can optimize testosterone levels, improve muscle growth, and maintain long-term health and vitality.

CHAPTER 5

MANAGING CORTISOL & STRESS

How Chronic Stress Disrupts Muscle Growth and Fat Metabolism

Cortisol, often referred to as the "stress hormone," is essential in small amounts for energy regulation and immune function. However, when cortisol levels remain elevated due to chronic stress, it negatively impacts metabolism, muscle growth, and fat storage.

The Effects of Chronic Stress on the Body

- **Muscle Breakdown:** Cortisol breaks down muscle protein into amino acids, reducing muscle mass over time.

- **Increased Fat Storage:** High cortisol levels signal the body to store fat, particularly around the abdominal area.

- **Slower Recovery:** Elevated stress hormones reduce the body's ability to repair muscle tissue after workouts.

> **Disrupted Sleep Patterns:** Poor sleep due to stress leads to further hormonal imbalances and fatigue.

> **Weakened Immune System:** Chronic stress weakens immune function, making the body more susceptible to illness.

To counteract these effects, managing stress through lifestyle changes is essential for maintaining long-term health and fitness.

The Benefits of Yoga, Meditation, and Sleep

Yoga for Cortisol Management

Yoga has been scientifically proven to reduce cortisol levels, improve flexibility, and promote relaxation. Regular practice helps manage stress, leading to better hormonal balance and improved recovery after workouts.

Best Yoga Poses for Stress Reduction

> **Child's Pose (Balasana):** Helps release tension and calms the nervous system.

> **Forward Bend (Uttanasana):** Stimulates blood flow and reduces anxiety.

> **Corpse Pose (Savasana):** Promotes deep relaxation and stress relief.

Meditation for Hormonal Balance

Meditation helps activate the parasympathetic nervous system, lowering stress levels and promoting mindfulness. Deep breathing exercises (Pranayama) are particularly effective in regulating cortisol.

Techniques to Try

> **Mindfulness Meditation:** Focuses on being present and reducing negative thoughts.

> **Breathwork (Anulom Vilom):** Balances the nervous system and enhances relaxation.

> **Guided Visualization:** Uses mental imagery to promote calmness and stress relief.

The Role of Sleep in Cortisol Regulation

Sleep plays a critical role in controlling cortisol levels and promoting muscle recovery. Poor sleep leads to an increase in stress hormones, which can negatively impact strength training results.

Tips for Better Sleep

- ➤ Stick to a consistent sleep schedule (7-9 hours per night).

- ➤ Avoid caffeine and screens at least one hour before bedtime.

- ➤ Create a relaxing bedtime routine with meditation or reading.

Exercise Modifications to Prevent Overtraining and Burnout

While exercise is beneficial for stress management, excessive training without adequate recovery can lead to overtraining syndrome (OTS), which increases cortisol levels and reduces performance.

Signs of Overtraining

- ➤ Persistent muscle soreness and fatigue.

- ➤ Increased irritability and restlessness.

- ➤ Weakened immune system and frequent illnesses.

- ➤ Decreased motivation and plateauing in progress.

How to Prevent Overtraining and Burnout

1. **Prioritize Recovery Days:**

   o   Incorporate at least one rest day per week.

   o   Use active recovery techniques like stretching, foam rolling, or light walking.

2. **Modify Workout Intensity:**

   o   Avoid excessive cardio and high-intensity training without sufficient recovery.

   o   Balance strength training with lower-impact exercises like swimming or cycling.

3. **Adjust Training Volume:**

   o   Train smarter, not harder. Short, high-quality workouts (45-60 minutes) are more effective than long, exhausting sessions.

4. **Incorporate Stress-Reducing Activities:**

   o   Engage in hobbies that promote relaxation, such as painting, gardening, or listening to music.

   o   Spend time in nature to lower cortisol levels naturally.

Final Takeaways: Achieving a Balanced Approach to Stress and Cortisol Management

- ➤ Chronic stress leads to hormonal imbalances that hinder muscle growth and promote fat gain.

- ➤ Yoga, meditation, and quality sleep are essential tools for reducing cortisol levels.

- ➤ Avoid overtraining by prioritizing recovery and modifying workout intensity.

- ➤ Engage in daily stress-relieving activities to maintain overall hormonal balance.

By implementing these stress management strategies, individuals can enhance their training performance, optimize hormone function, and achieve long-term physical and mental well-being.

CHAPTER 6

BALANCING ESTROGEN & TESTOSTERONE

Understanding Estrogen Dominance in Men and Women

Estrogen and testosterone are two of the most influential hormones affecting body composition, strength, and metabolism. While testosterone is more prominent in men and estrogen in women, both hormones are present in both sexes and must be balanced for optimal health.

What Is Estrogen Dominance?

Estrogen dominance occurs when estrogen levels are too high in relation to testosterone. This imbalance can happen in both men and women and is associated with weight gain, fatigue, mood swings, and increased fat storage.

Signs of Estrogen Dominance

> Increased fat accumulation, particularly around the hips and thighs.

> ➤ Mood swings, irritability, and low energy.

> ➤ Decreased muscle tone and strength.

> ➤ Water retention and bloating.

> ➤ Hormonal acne and skin issues.

For men, excess estrogen can contribute to gynecomastia (development of male breast tissue) and reduced libido. For women, it can lead to irregular menstrual cycles, PMS symptoms, and difficulty losing weight.

The Impact of Estrogen on Fat Distribution

Estrogen plays a crucial role in regulating fat storage. Women naturally have higher estrogen levels, which is why they store more fat in the hips, thighs, and buttocks, whereas men tend to store excess fat in the abdominal area.

However, excessive estrogen can lead to disproportionate fat distribution and make it harder to burn fat, particularly when combined with low testosterone levels.

Effects of High Estrogen Levels

> ➤ Increased fat retention in the lower body.

> ➤ Difficulty losing weight despite diet and exercise.

- Reduced muscle mass and strength.

- Increased risk of insulin resistance and metabolic disorders.

Natural Ways to Maintain Hormone Balance

Maintaining a balance between estrogen and testosterone is crucial for both men and women. This can be achieved through lifestyle modifications, diet, and proper exercise.

Strength Training for Hormonal Balance

Resistance training has been shown to naturally increase testosterone while helping regulate estrogen levels.

Best Exercises for Balancing Hormones

- **Squats and Deadlifts:** These compound movements activate large muscle groups, promoting testosterone production.

- **High-Intensity Interval Training (HIIT):** Short bursts of intense activity followed by rest improve insulin sensitivity and reduce estrogen dominance.

> ➤ **Upper Body Strength Training:** Exercises like bench presses, rows, and pull-ups enhance muscle growth and support testosterone production.

Nutritional Strategies to Reduce Estrogen Dominance

A well-balanced diet can help regulate estrogen and testosterone levels. Certain foods support hormone detoxification, while others may contribute to hormonal imbalances.

Foods to Support Estrogen Detoxification

> ➤ **Cruciferous Vegetables:** Broccoli, cauliflower, kale, and cabbage contain compounds that help the liver break down excess estrogen.

> ➤ **Flaxseeds and Chia Seeds:** Rich in fiber and omega-3s, these seeds aid in estrogen metabolism.

> ➤ **Turmeric and Ginger:** Known for their anti-inflammatory properties, they support liver function and hormone balance.

Foods to Increase Testosterone Naturally

> ➤ **Healthy Fats:** Nuts, seeds, olive oil, and ghee are essential for hormone production.

> **Protein Sources:** Lean meats, eggs, paneer, and legumes support muscle maintenance and testosterone production.

> **Zinc-Rich Foods:** Pumpkin seeds, almonds, and chickpeas boost testosterone synthesis.

Foods to Avoid

> **Processed Foods and Sugars:** These disrupt insulin levels and contribute to hormonal imbalances.

> **Soy-Based Products:** Excess soy intake may increase estrogen levels.

> **Alcohol and Caffeine:** These can interfere with liver detoxification and hormone metabolism.

The Role of Sleep and Stress Management in Hormonal Balance

Poor sleep and chronic stress elevate cortisol levels, which can suppress testosterone and increase estrogen dominance.

Ways to Optimize Sleep and Reduce Stress

> **Prioritize Deep Sleep:** Aim for 7-9 hours per night to allow proper hormone regulation.

> **Practice Meditation and Yoga:** Stress reduction techniques help lower cortisol and keep estrogen levels in check.

> **Engage in Outdoor Activities:** Exposure to sunlight helps boost testosterone through vitamin D synthesis.

Final Takeaways: Achieving Estrogen-Testosterone Balance Naturally

> Strength training is essential for maintaining healthy testosterone levels and regulating estrogen.

> Eating a nutrient-dense diet with a focus on whole foods supports hormonal detoxification.

> Managing stress and prioritizing sleep are crucial for preventing estrogen dominance.

> Avoiding processed foods and excess soy intake can help maintain an optimal hormonal balance.

By following these strategies, individuals can achieve a healthier, stronger body while minimizing the negative effects of estrogen dominance and low testosterone.

CHAPTER 7

STRENGTH TRAINING & INSULIN SENSITIVITY

How Lifting Weights Improves Glucose Metabolism

Insulin is a hormone responsible for regulating blood sugar levels. Poor insulin sensitivity, or insulin resistance, can lead to conditions such as obesity, Type 2 diabetes, and metabolic syndrome. Strength training is one of the most effective natural strategies to improve insulin sensitivity and optimize glucose metabolism.

Effects of Strength Training on Glucose Metabolism

> **Increases Muscle Mass:** Muscle tissue absorbs glucose for energy, reducing excess blood sugar levels.

> **Enhances Insulin Sensitivity:** Lifting weights makes muscle cells more responsive to insulin, reducing the risk of diabetes.

> ➤ **Reduces Visceral Fat:** Strength training helps burn fat around internal organs, improving metabolic health.

> ➤ **Boosts Mitochondrial Function:** Strength workouts enhance cellular energy production, aiding glucose utilization.

Exercise and Dietary Strategies to Prevent Diabetes

Diabetes prevention is a key aspect of hormonal health, and combining exercise with proper nutrition can significantly reduce the risk of insulin resistance.

Best Strength Training Exercises for Insulin Sensitivity

1. **Compound Movements:**

   - Squats, deadlifts, and lunges activate large muscle groups and improve glucose uptake.

   - Bench presses and pull-ups stimulate upper body muscles, enhancing insulin efficiency.

2. **High-Intensity Interval Training (HIIT):**

   - Short bursts of intense exercise followed by rest periods enhance insulin sensitivity.

o   Example: Sprint for 30 seconds, rest for 60 seconds, repeat for 15 minutes.

3. **Progressive Overload Training:**

o   Gradually increasing weight over time challenges muscles, improving glucose metabolism.

o   Perform 8-12 reps of moderate-to-heavy weightlifting per set.

Dietary Adjustments for Blood Sugar Control

1. **Increase Fiber Intake:**

o   Vegetables, whole grains, and legumes slow glucose absorption.

2. **Prioritize Lean Proteins:**

o   Chicken, fish, eggs, and tofu stabilize blood sugar levels.

3. **Healthy Fats for Hormonal Balance:**

o   Nuts, seeds, and olive oil prevent insulin spikes.

4. **Reduce Processed Carbohydrates:**

o   Avoid white bread, sugary drinks, and processed snacks.

The Benefits of Intermittent Fasting for Hormonal Health

Intermittent fasting (IF) has gained popularity as a strategy for improving insulin sensitivity, balancing hormones, and promoting overall metabolic health.

How IF Improves Insulin Sensitivity

> **Reduces Fasting Blood Sugar:** Periodic fasting allows insulin levels to drop, making cells more responsive.

> **Enhances Fat Burning:** Fasting forces the body to use stored fat for energy, reducing insulin resistance.

> **Promotes Cellular Repair:** IF triggers autophagy, the body's natural detoxification process.

Popular Intermittent Fasting Methods

1. **16:8 Method:**

   o Fast for 16 hours, eat within an 8-hour window.

   o Suitable for beginners and those seeking gradual benefits.

2. **5:2 Diet:**

   o Eat normally for five days, restrict calories to 500-600 for two days.

3. **Alternate-Day Fasting:**

   o Fasting every other day to optimize insulin regulation.

Combining IF with Strength Training

> **Train in a Fasted State:** Workouts before the first meal may enhance fat oxidation.

> **Break the Fast with Protein:** Consuming protein post-workout supports muscle recovery and glucose regulation.

> **Hydration is Key:** Drinking water, black coffee, or green tea helps sustain energy levels during fasting periods.

Final Takeaways: Achieving Insulin Balance Through Strength Training & Nutrition

> Strength training is one of the most effective ways to enhance insulin sensitivity and prevent diabetes.

> ➤ Compound exercises, HIIT, and progressive overload improve glucose metabolism and fat loss.

> ➤ A diet rich in fiber, protein, and healthy fats supports blood sugar control.

> ➤ Intermittent fasting is a powerful tool to regulate insulin, promote fat loss, and enhance overall metabolic health.

By integrating these strategies into daily life, individuals can optimize insulin function, improve energy levels, and prevent metabolic diseases naturally.

THYROID HEALTH & ENERGY REGULATION

The Thyroid's Role in Metabolism and Fat Loss

The thyroid gland, located in the neck, plays a crucial role in metabolism, energy production, and fat loss. It produces two primary hormones—**thyroxine (T4) and triiodothyronine (T3)**—which regulate metabolic rate and influence how the body utilizes energy.

Effects of Thyroid Dysfunction on Health

> **Hypothyroidism (Underactive Thyroid):** Leads to weight gain, fatigue, sluggish metabolism, and cold intolerance.

> **Hyperthyroidism (Overactive Thyroid):** Results in rapid weight loss, increased heart rate, anxiety, and excessive sweating.

> ➤ **Hashimoto's Disease:** An autoimmune disorder that causes inflammation of the thyroid gland, leading to hypothyroidism.

A well-functioning thyroid is essential for maintaining a healthy weight, muscle growth, and energy levels. Ensuring optimal thyroid function through strength training and proper nutrition can help regulate metabolism and prevent thyroid-related disorders.

How Strength Training Supports Thyroid Function

Strength training offers multiple benefits for thyroid health by boosting metabolism, regulating hormones, and improving overall energy levels.

Benefits of Strength Training for Thyroid Health

1. **Increases Resting Metabolic Rate (RMR):**

   o Resistance training helps build lean muscle, which requires more energy to maintain, leading to a higher metabolic rate.

2. **Enhances Insulin Sensitivity:**

   o Strength training reduces insulin resistance, a common issue in people with hypothyroidism.

3. **Stimulates Thyroid Hormone Production:**

   o   Regular resistance exercise encourages T3 and T4 production, optimizing metabolism.

4. **Reduces Inflammation and Autoimmune Response:**

   o   Exercise lowers inflammation, which can benefit those with autoimmune thyroid conditions like Hashimoto's.

Best Strength Training Exercises for Thyroid Health

   ➤ **Compound Movements:** Squats, deadlifts, and lunges stimulate muscle growth and metabolism.

   ➤ **Resistance Band Workouts:** Provide controlled movements that help regulate hormones.

   ➤ **Core Strength Exercises:** Planks and leg raises stabilize energy levels and improve posture.

   ➤ **High-Intensity Interval Training (HIIT):** Short bursts of intense exercise followed by recovery enhance metabolic function.

Nutritional Guidelines for Maintaining a Healthy Thyroid

Diet plays a critical role in thyroid health. Certain nutrients support thyroid hormone production, while others can disrupt it.

Essential Nutrients for Thyroid Health

1. **Iodine:**

   - Found in **iodized salt, seaweed, fish, and dairy**.

   - Essential for producing T3 and T4 hormones.

2. **Selenium:**

   - Found in **Brazil nuts, eggs, sunflower seeds, and mushrooms**.

   - Helps convert T4 into its active form, T3.

3. **Zinc:**

   - Found in **pumpkin seeds, almonds, lentils, and lean meats**.

   - Supports immune function and thyroid hormone production.

4. **Iron:**

   o Found in **spinach, legumes, and red meat**.

   o Important for proper thyroid function and oxygen transport.

5. **Vitamin D:**

   o Found in **fortified dairy, fish, and sunlight exposure**.

   o Crucial for immune health and inflammation control.

Foods to Avoid for Thyroid Health

   ➤ **Processed Foods & Sugary Beverages:** Cause insulin resistance and hormonal imbalances.

   ➤ **Excess Soy Products:** Interfere with thyroid hormone absorption.

   ➤ **Gluten (for some individuals with Hashimoto's):** Can trigger inflammation in people with autoimmune thyroid conditions.

   ➤ **Excess Cruciferous Vegetables (if iodine deficient):** Large amounts of raw broccoli, cabbage, and kale can interfere with iodine absorption.

Lifestyle Changes to Improve Thyroid Function

In addition to strength training and nutrition, certain lifestyle modifications can further support thyroid health.

1. **Manage Stress Effectively:**

    ➤ Chronic stress increases cortisol, which can suppress thyroid function.

    ➤ Practice yoga, meditation, and deep breathing exercises to manage stress.

2. **Get Quality Sleep:**

    ➤ Sleep deprivation disrupts hormone production, leading to fatigue and weight gain.

    ➤ Aim for 7-9 hours of quality sleep each night.

3. **Reduce Exposure to Toxins:**

    ➤ Avoid endocrine-disrupting chemicals (EDCs) found in plastics and non-stick cookware.

    ➤ Opt for glass or stainless steel food storage containers.

4. Stay Hydrated:

> Dehydration affects metabolism and energy levels.

> Drink at least 2-3 liters of water per day to support thyroid function.

Final Takeaways: Optimizing Thyroid Health Through Strength Training & Nutrition

> The thyroid plays a critical role in metabolism, energy production, and fat loss.

> Strength training boosts thyroid hormone production and improves insulin sensitivity.

> A diet rich in iodine, selenium, zinc, and vitamin D supports optimal thyroid function.

> Managing stress, sleep, and reducing toxin exposure further enhances thyroid health.

By following these strategies, individuals can maintain a healthy thyroid, optimize energy levels, and support long-term metabolic health.

CHAPTER 9

CREATING AN EFFECTIVE TRAINING PLAN

A well-structured training plan is crucial for achieving fitness goals, improving strength, and maintaining long-term health. As we age, a carefully planned resistance training program helps maintain muscle mass, joint health, and overall well-being. This chapter focuses on key resistance exercises for aging adults, progressing safely in strength training, and adjusting workouts based on age and experience.

Key Resistance Exercises for Aging Adults

Resistance exercises should be tailored to improve strength, mobility, and endurance while minimizing the risk of injury. The following exercises are fundamental for older adults:

1. **Lower Body Strength**

   ➤ **Squats (Bodyweight, Goblet, or Assisted Squats)** – Build leg strength and improve balance.

> **Lunges (Forward or Reverse)** – Strengthen the lower body and enhance coordination.

> **Leg Press Machine** – Provides controlled resistance to maintain leg strength.

> **Calf Raises** – Improve ankle stability and prevent falls.

2. **Upper Body Strength**

> **Push-Ups (Wall or Inclined Variations for Beginners)** – Strengthen the chest, shoulders, and arms.

> **Dumbbell Shoulder Press** – Builds shoulder strength and stability.

> **Seated Row (Cable or Resistance Bands)** – Improves posture and back strength.

> **Bicep Curls and Triceps Dips** – Help maintain arm strength and function.

3. **Core Stability**

> **Planks (Modified or Full)** – Strengthen core muscles for improved posture and balance.

> **Dead Bug Exercise** – Enhances coordination and stability.

➤ **Russian Twists (With or Without Weights)** – Improve core strength and flexibility.

4. **Functional Movements**

➤ **Hip Bridges** – Improve lower back strength and glute activation.

➤ **Step-Ups (With or Without Dumbbells)** – Enhance leg endurance and coordination.

➤ **Seated to Standing Exercises** – Mimic real-life movements to build strength.

How to Progress in Strength Training Safely

Strength training should be progressive to ensure steady improvements while minimizing injury risk. Here's how to safely progress:

1. **Start with Low Resistance and Increase Gradually**

➤ Begin with bodyweight exercises before incorporating resistance bands or light weights.

➤ Gradually increase resistance by 5-10% every few weeks based on strength gains.

2. Prioritize Form Over Weight

- ➤ Proper technique prevents injuries and ensures muscle engagement.

- ➤ Use mirrors or work with a coach to maintain correct posture.

3. Increase Repetitions and Sets Gradually

- ➤ Start with **2-3 sets of 10-12 repetitions** and increa0se as strength improves.

- ➤ Progress to **3-4 sets of 8-10 reps** with moderate weight for muscle building.

4. Allow Sufficient Recovery Time

- ➤ Train each muscle group **2-3 times per week** with rest days in between.

- ➤ Recovery is crucial for muscle repair and long-term progress.

Adjusting Workouts Based on Age and Experience

As individuals age, training plans should be adapted to prevent injury and ensure sustainable progress.

1. **Adapting to Experience Level**

   ➤ **Beginners:** Start with low-impact, bodyweight exercises and focus on mobility.

   ➤ **Intermediate Lifters:** Gradually introduce resistance and compound movements.

   ➤ **Advanced Lifters:** Incorporate heavier weights and higher training volume with adequate recovery.

2. **Addressing Joint Health and Mobility**

   ➤ Include mobility exercises to reduce stiffness and improve movement patterns.

   ➤ Modify movements (e.g., chair-assisted squats, resistance bands instead of free weights).

3. **Incorporating Cardiovascular and Flexibility Training**

   ➤ Combine **strength training with walking, swimming, or cycling** to support heart health.

   ➤ **Yoga and stretching** improve flexibility and reduce the risk of injury.

Final Takeaways: Building a Sustainable Strength Training Routine

- Strength training enhances muscle function, metabolic health, and longevity.

- A well-balanced routine includes **lower body, upper body, core, and functional movements**.

- Gradually increasing resistance and focusing on form ensures **safe and effective progression**.

- Adjusting training plans based on age and experience helps maintain long-term fitness goals.

- Recovery, mobility, and flexibility exercises are key to **injury prevention and sustained health**.

By incorporating these principles into a structured routine, individuals can achieve long-term strength, resilience, and independence as they age.

CHAPTER 10

NUTRITION FOR STRENGTH & HORMONAL BALANCE

A well-structured diet plays a fundamental role in building muscle, optimizing hormonal balance, and ensuring longevity. For strength training to be effective, it must be supported by proper nutrition, particularly protein intake, micronutrients, and an overall balanced Indian diet.

Best Protein Sources in an Indian Diet

Protein is essential for muscle recovery, strength, and hormonal balance. Indian diets, often being plant-based or vegetarian, can sometimes lack sufficient protein. However, by choosing the right sources, one can ensure optimal protein intake.

1. **Animal-Based Protein Sources**

   ➤ **Eggs:** A complete protein source rich in essential amino acids, vitamin B12, and choline.

   ➤ **Chicken and Fish:** Lean proteins that help in muscle growth and repair.

➢ **Dairy Products:** Paneer, curd, and milk provide high-quality casein and whey protein for sustained muscle recovery.

2. Plant-Based Protein Sources

➢ **Lentils (Dal):** A staple in Indian households, offering protein and fiber for digestion.

➢ **Chickpeas and Black Beans:** Excellent sources of plant protein, fiber, and iron.

➢ **Soy Products (Tofu & Tempeh):** High in protein and contains phytoestrogens that support hormonal health.

➢ **Nuts & Seeds (Almonds, Pumpkin Seeds, Flaxseeds):** Offer plant-based protein along with healthy fats.

3. Protein-Rich Grains and Other Sources

➢ **Quinoa & Millets:** High in protein and fiber, perfect substitutes for refined grains.

➢ **Greek Yogurt:** Packed with probiotics and protein to aid digestion and muscle recovery.

➢ **Protein Powders (Whey & Plant-Based):** Can be supplemented to meet daily protein needs, especially for vegetarians.

The Role of Micronutrients in Muscle Recovery

Micronutrients are as crucial as macronutrients in strength training and hormonal balance. Deficiencies can lead to poor recovery, muscle fatigue, and slow progress.

1. **Essential Vitamins for Strength Training**

   - **Vitamin D:** Supports bone strength and testosterone production; best sources are sunlight, fortified dairy, and eggs.

   - **Vitamin B12:** Crucial for energy metabolism and nerve function, found in dairy, eggs, and fish.

   - **Vitamin C:** Aids in collagen synthesis and muscle repair; found in citrus fruits and bell peppers.

2. **Essential Minerals for Muscle Function**

   - **Magnesium:** Helps with muscle relaxation and recovery; sources include spinach, nuts, and bananas.

   - **Zinc:** Supports testosterone levels and immune function; found in pumpkin seeds and dairy.

> **Iron:** Prevents fatigue and supports oxygen transport in the body; found in lentils and leafy greens.

How Traditional Indian Diets Can Be Optimized for Longevity

The Indian diet is rich in complex carbohydrates, fiber, and essential spices. However, modern dietary habits have introduced excessive processed foods, leading to metabolic issues. By making small adjustments, one can ensure longevity and optimal health.

1. **Balancing Carbohydrates for Energy**

   > Replace refined grains (white rice, maida) with whole grains like **brown rice, millets, and quinoa**.

   > Include fiber-rich foods such as **vegetables, fruits, and legumes** to slow digestion and maintain energy levels.

2. **Healthy Fats for Hormonal Balance**

   > Include **ghee, coconut oil, and nuts** for hormone production and metabolism.

   > Avoid trans fats found in processed and fried foods.

3. Importance of Hydration

➤ Drink **3-4 liters of water daily** to support digestion, nutrient transport, and muscle function.

➤ Herbal teas like **green tea and ashwagandha tea** aid in detoxification and relaxation.

4. Optimizing Meal Timing for Strength and Hormones

➤ **Pre-Workout Nutrition:** A combination of carbs and protein (banana with peanut butter, oats with yogurt) enhances workout performance.

➤ **Post-Workout Nutrition:** Protein-rich meals like **dal-rice, paneer with roti, or eggs with toast** ensure muscle repair.

➤ **Intermittent Fasting:** Can be an effective strategy to regulate insulin levels and optimize fat metabolism.

Final Takeaways: Achieving Strength & Hormonal Balance Through Nutrition

➤ Prioritize **protein intake** with a mix of animal and plant-based sources.

➤ Ensure adequate **micronutrient consumption** for optimal muscle recovery.

> Optimize **traditional Indian diets** by balancing carbohydrates, incorporating healthy fats, and staying hydrated.

> Align meal timing with training goals to maximize muscle growth and hormonal balance.

By following these nutritional principles, individuals can enhance their strength, improve hormonal health, and promote longevity while enjoying an Indian diet tailored for fitness and wellness.

CHAPTER 11

DEBUNKING STRENGTH TRAINING MYTHS

Strength training is often misunderstood due to myths and misinformation. Many people believe it is only for bodybuilders, that lifting heavy weights makes women bulky, or that older adults should avoid resistance training. In reality, strength training benefits people of all ages and fitness levels. This chapter addresses these misconceptions and explains why strength training is a key component of long-term health and vitality.

Myth #1: Strength Training Is Only for Bodybuilders

Many believe that strength training is reserved for bodybuilders who want to achieve a highly muscular physique. However, this could not be further from the truth. Strength training offers a wide range of benefits beyond muscle size:

1. **Improves Functional Strength**

   - Lifting weights enhances overall strength, making daily activities like carrying groceries, climbing stairs, and lifting objects easier.

   - Strength training reduces the risk of injuries by improving joint stability and posture.

2. **Boosts Metabolism and Fat Loss**

   - More muscle mass increases resting metabolic rate, meaning the body burns more calories even at rest.

   - Strength training helps maintain lean muscle while reducing body fat.

3. **Supports Cardiovascular Health**

   - Resistance training improves heart health by lowering blood pressure and improving circulation.

   - It reduces the risk of chronic diseases such as diabetes and obesity.

Myth #2: Lifting Heavy Weights Makes Women Bulky

A common fear among women is that lifting weights will make them appear overly muscular or bulky. In reality, women have lower testosterone levels than men, making it difficult to develop large muscles naturally. Instead, strength training helps women achieve a toned, lean, and strong physique.

1. **Promotes a Toned Body**

   ➤ Resistance training increases muscle definition without excessive bulk.

   ➤ It helps shape the body by enhancing lean muscle mass while reducing fat.

2. **Strengthens Bones and Prevents Osteoporosis**

   ➤ Women are at a higher risk of osteoporosis as they age. Strength training increases bone density, reducing fracture risk.

   ➤ Exercises like squats, lunges, and deadlifts strengthen bones and joints.

3. **Enhances Hormonal Balance**

   ➤ Strength training improves insulin sensitivity, reducing the risk of hormonal imbalances.

> It helps regulate estrogen levels, preventing weight gain and mood swings.

Myth #3: Older Adults Should Avoid Strength Training

Another widespread misconception is that older adults should avoid strength training due to the risk of injury. However, resistance training is one of the most effective ways for aging individuals to maintain mobility, strength, and independence.

1. **Prevents Age-Related Muscle Loss (Sarcopenia)**

   > After age 30, muscle mass naturally declines. Strength training preserves muscle strength and function.

   > Lifting weights improves balance and reduces the risk of falls.

2. **Supports Joint Health and Reduces Pain**

   > Contrary to belief, strength training can **relieve joint pain** by strengthening the muscles that support joints.

   > Low-impact resistance exercises help individuals with arthritis and chronic pain.

3. Improves Cognitive Function

> ➤ Studies show that strength training improves memory, focus, and mental sharpness in older adults.

> ➤ Exercise releases endorphins, reducing stress and enhancing overall mood.

Practical Steps to Overcome Strength Training Myths

Now that we have debunked these common myths, let's discuss how individuals of all ages and fitness levels can incorporate strength training into their lives:

1. Start with Bodyweight Exercises

> ➤ Push-ups, squats, lunges, and planks are great beginner exercises that build strength safely.

> ➤ Resistance bands can be used for additional support and progression.

2. Gradually Add Resistance

> ➤ Start with light weights and gradually increase resistance as strength improves.

> ➤ Focus on proper form rather than lifting heavy weights initially.

3. Customize Workouts for Individual Needs

- ➤ Strength training programs should be adjusted based on fitness level, age, and personal goals.

- ➤ Older adults can opt for seated or modified strength exercises to accommodate mobility limitations.

Final Takeaways: Embracing Strength Training for Everyone

- ➤ Strength training is not just for bodybuilders; it benefits people of all ages and fitness levels.

- ➤ Women will not become bulky from lifting weights but will instead develop a lean, strong physique.

- ➤ Older adults can safely engage in resistance training to maintain mobility, prevent muscle loss, and improve bone health.

- ➤ With proper technique, gradual progression, and consistency, strength training can be an essential part of lifelong health and wellness.

By overcoming these myths, individuals can embrace strength training confidently, improving their overall health, strength, and vitality.

CHAPTER 12

SUPPLEMENTS & NATURAL ADAPTOGENS

In addition to a well-balanced diet and strength training, certain supplements and natural adaptogens can support muscle growth, recovery, and hormonal health. India has a rich history of using herbal remedies for wellness, and modern research has confirmed the benefits of many traditional herbs in supporting physical performance and recovery.

Indian Herbs Like Ashwagandha and Shatavari for Hormone Support

1. **Ashwagandha: The Stress-Reducing Powerhouse**

   ➤ An adaptogenic herb known for reducing cortisol levels and managing stress.

   ➤ Enhances testosterone production, which aids in muscle growth and recovery.

   ➤ Improves endurance, strength, and mental focus, making it an excellent supplement for athletes.

- Best consumed as **capsules, powder mixed with warm milk, or tea**.

2. **Shatavari: The Female Hormone Balancer**

- Traditionally used for balancing estrogen and improving reproductive health in women.

- Supports endurance and muscle recovery, making it beneficial for women involved in strength training.

- Enhances immunity and overall energy levels.

- Consumed as **capsules, tea, or mixed with milk**.

3. **Safed Musli: Natural Testosterone Booster**

- Known for enhancing libido and testosterone levels in men.

- Improves muscle recovery and endurance.

- Often used in Ayurvedic formulations to support muscle-building and vitality.

4. **Gokshura (Tribulus Terrestris): Performance Enhancer**

- Helps boost natural testosterone production.

➢ Increases energy and endurance, making it beneficial for strength athletes.

➢ Used in Ayurvedic medicine for muscle recovery and kidney health.

Best Supplements for Muscle Growth and Recovery

1. **Whey Protein: The Foundation of Muscle Growth**

➢ One of the most easily digestible and fast-absorbing protein sources.

➢ Helps repair and build muscle tissue after strength training.

➢ Comes in various forms: **concentrate, isolate, and hydrolysate**.

➢ Ideal consumption: **Post-workout in shakes or smoothies**.

2. **Creatine Monohydrate: The Strength Booster**

➢ Increases energy production in muscles, leading to improved strength and endurance.

➢ Helps with muscle hydration and promotes lean muscle mass.

> Recommended dosage: **3-5 grams per day, preferably post-workout**.

3. Branched-Chain Amino Acids (BCAAs): Recovery and Endurance

> Contains leucine, isoleucine, and valine, which aid in muscle recovery and reduce muscle soreness.

> Prevents muscle breakdown during intense workouts.

> Best taken **pre-workout or intra-workout for muscle endurance**.

4. Omega-3 Fatty Acids: Joint and Muscle Recovery

> Reduces inflammation, helping with muscle recovery.

> Supports heart health and cognitive function.

> Found in **fatty fish, flaxseeds, and fish oil capsules**.

5. Vitamin D & Magnesium: Essential for Strength

> Vitamin D is crucial for bone health and testosterone regulation.

> ➤ Magnesium helps with muscle relaxation and prevents cramps.

> ➤ Found in **fortified dairy, nuts, leafy greens, and supplements**.

How to Use Supplements Safely and Effectively

1. **Understand Your Needs**

> ➤ Supplements should complement a **well-balanced diet**, not replace it.

> ➤ Choose supplements based on individual fitness goals (muscle gain, endurance, recovery).

2. **Dosage and Timing Matters**

> ➤ Protein: **Post-workout for muscle repair**.

> ➤ Creatine: **Daily for strength and endurance**.

> ➤ BCAAs: **Pre or intra-workout for muscle preservation**.

> ➤ Ashwagandha: **Before bedtime to lower cortisol and enhance recovery**.

3. Choose High-Quality Supplements

- ➢ Look for **third-party tested supplements** to ensure purity and efficacy.

- ➢ Avoid supplements with artificial additives, excessive sugar, or fillers.

4. Monitor Your Body's Response

- ➢ Track how your body responds to different supplements.

- ➢ If any adverse effects occur, discontinue use and consult a nutritionist.

Final Takeaways: Optimizing Strength Training with Supplements & Adaptogens

- ➢ Indian herbs like **Ashwagandha, Shatavari, Safed Musli, and Gokshura** support hormonal balance and muscle recovery.

- ➢ **Whey protein, creatine, BCAAs, and omega-3s** help improve strength and endurance.

- ➢ Supplements should be used **alongside a well-balanced diet** and not as a substitute.

> ➢ Choosing high-quality supplements and monitoring intake ensures **safety and effectiveness**.

By integrating **natural adaptogens and essential supplements**, individuals can enhance strength, endurance, and recovery, ultimately achieving long-term fitness and hormonal balance.

CHAPTER 13

RECOVERY & REGENERATION

Why Rest and Recovery Are as Important as Training

Strength training stimulates muscle growth, but true progress happens during the recovery phase. Recovery allows muscles to rebuild stronger, prevents injuries, and ensures long-term sustainability in fitness routines.

1. Muscle Repair and Growth

- When you lift weights, small tears form in the muscle fibers. These tears need time to repair and grow stronger.

- Without adequate recovery, muscle breakdown can exceed muscle building, leading to stagnation or even muscle loss.

2. Preventing Overtraining Syndrome

- Overtraining can cause fatigue, irritability, weakened immunity, and even injuries.

- ➤ Symptoms include prolonged muscle soreness, trouble sleeping, and decreased performance.

- ➤ Structured rest periods help prevent burnout and ensure consistent progress.

3. Optimizing Hormone Levels

- ➤ Training stresses the body and elevates cortisol. Recovery helps bring these stress hormones back to normal.

- ➤ Rest promotes the release of **growth hormone and testosterone**, both critical for muscle repair and strength gains.

The Benefits of Massage, Stretching, and Active Recovery

Proper recovery isn't just about taking complete rest days. Techniques like massage, stretching, and active recovery improve circulation, reduce muscle stiffness, and aid in faster healing.

1. Massage Therapy for Muscle Recovery

- ➤ Deep tissue and sports massages break down knots and increase blood flow to sore muscles.

- ➤ Reduces **inflammation** and flushes out metabolic waste from training.

- ➤ Can be done professionally or through self-massage tools like **foam rollers and massage guns**.

2. The Importance of Stretching

- ➤ Stretching improves flexibility, enhances muscle function, and prevents injuries.

- ➤ Best performed **after workouts** to lengthen muscles and improve range of motion.

- ➤ Types of stretching:

  - ○ **Static Stretching** (holding a stretch for 15-30 seconds)

  - ○ **Dynamic Stretching** (controlled movements that prepare the muscles for activity)

3. Active Recovery for Long-Term Strength

- ➤ Light activities such as walking, swimming, and yoga keep blood flowing without stressing the muscles.

- ➤ Helps **reduce stiffness** and promotes mobility.

- ➤ Active recovery days should be included at least **once or twice a week** to prevent stagnation.

How Sleep Influences Hormone Balance and Muscle Repair

Sleep is the body's most powerful recovery tool. Poor sleep can sabotage muscle growth, increase cortisol, and lead to weight gain.

1. **Growth Hormone Production**

    ➤ The majority of growth hormone is released during **deep sleep**.

    ➤ This hormone is crucial for tissue repair, fat loss, and overall recovery.

2. **Testosterone and Muscle Repair**

    ➤ Sleep plays a key role in regulating **testosterone levels**.

    ➤ Low testosterone leads to **muscle weakness, fat gain, and poor recovery**.

3. **Cortisol Reduction and Stress Management**

    ➤ Poor sleep elevates cortisol, leading to **fat gain and muscle breakdown**.

    ➤ Deep sleep balances cortisol and ensures optimal recovery.

4. **How to Improve Sleep for Better Recovery**

- **Maintain a Consistent Sleep Schedule** – Aim for **7-9 hours of sleep per night**.

- **Limit Blue Light Exposure** – Avoid screens at least **one hour before bed**.

- **Optimize Your Sleep Environment** – Keep the room **cool, dark, and quiet**.

- **Use Relaxation Techniques** – Meditation, breathing exercises, and herbal teas (such as chamomile) help with relaxation.

Final Takeaways: Prioritizing Recovery for Strength and Longevity

- Recovery is **just as important as training** in strength-building and longevity.

- **Massage, stretching, and active recovery** help improve flexibility, reduce stiffness, and speed up muscle healing.

- **Sleep is the ultimate recovery tool**, optimizing growth hormone and testosterone while reducing cortisol.

> ➤ **Properly scheduled rest days** prevent injuries, fatigue, and overtraining.

> ➤ A well-balanced approach to **training and recovery** ensures consistent strength gains and long-term wellness.

By incorporating **restorative techniques, proper sleep, and active recovery**, individuals can maximize their muscle gains, optimize hormonal health, and sustain long-term fitness.

CHAPTER 14

STRENGTH TRAINING & HORMONAL HEALTH IN INDIA

The Impact of Indian Dietary Habits and Cultural Perceptions

India has a diverse food culture that varies by region, religion, and tradition. While Indian diets are rich in whole foods, some habits may hinder strength training and hormonal balance.

1. **Vegetarianism and Protein Deficiency**

   ➢ A large portion of Indians follow a vegetarian diet, which can make it difficult to get complete proteins for muscle growth.

   ➢ Solutions: **Include lentils, dairy, quinoa, soy, nuts, and seeds to balance protein intake.**

2. **High Carbohydrate Consumption**

   ➢ Indian meals often focus on rice, chapatis, and potatoes, which can lead to insulin resistance when consumed in excess.

> ➢ Solutions: **Balance carb intake with high-fiber foods, vegetables, and protein sources.**

3. **Cooking Methods and Nutrient Loss**

> ➢ Overcooking vegetables and excessive frying can lead to loss of essential vitamins and minerals.

> ➢ Solutions: **Adopt steaming, roasting, and sautéing for nutrient retention.**

4. **Cultural Perceptions on Body Types and Fitness**

> ➢ Strength training is often associated with bodybuilding, leading to a lack of participation from women and older adults.

> ➢ Solution: **Educate the community about the benefits of strength training for all age groups.**

Overcoming Lifestyle Challenges to Build Strength

Modern Indian lifestyles involve long work hours, sedentary habits, and a lack of awareness about fitness. Strength training must be integrated into daily life to ensure long-term health benefits.

1. **Making Time for Strength Training**

   - Many people struggle with finding time to work out.

   - Solution: **Short, high-intensity workouts (20-30 minutes) can be effective for busy professionals.**

2. **Family and Social Expectations**

   - Women are often expected to focus on household responsibilities, leaving little time for fitness.

   - Solution: **Encourage fitness as a family activity and break stereotypes about women and strength training.**

3. **Access to Gyms and Equipment**

   - Many smaller towns lack proper fitness facilities.

   - Solution: **Home workouts using resistance bands, bodyweight exercises, and small weights can be just as effective.**

4. **Age-Related Concerns**

   - Older adults may hesitate to engage in strength training due to fear of injury.

> ➤ Solution: **Provide structured programs focusing on low-impact resistance exercises.**

Making Fitness a Long-Term Priority in Indian Households

To create a long-term fitness culture in India, strength training must be seen as a regular part of life, not just an occasional activity.

1. **Educating the Next Generation**

   > ➤ Schools should introduce basic strength training concepts alongside yoga and physical activity.

   > ➤ Parents must set an example by engaging in fitness routines.

2. **Strength Training for Families**

   > ➤ Engaging in activities like **group workouts, outdoor sports, and yoga** makes fitness a social bonding experience.

   > ➤ Traditional Indian activities like **kabaddi, wrestling, and martial arts** provide natural strength training benefits.

3. **Creating Supportive Communities**

   > ➤ Local fitness groups, walking clubs, and community gyms can encourage participation.

> Social media and online fitness challenges help build motivation and consistency.

4. Government and Workplace Initiatives

> More companies should introduce wellness programs, providing employees with gym access and health benefits.

> Government-led initiatives can promote fitness awareness campaigns, similar to Yoga Day initiatives.

Final Takeaways: Strength Training as a Lifelong Practice in India

> Indian diets must be optimized for strength by balancing **protein, carbs, and fats.**

> Overcoming cultural and lifestyle challenges is essential for making fitness accessible to everyone.

> Strength training should be embraced by **women, seniors, and young adults** alike for long-term health benefits.

> Schools, workplaces, and community centers should promote **strength training awareness.**

> ➤ **Fitness should be seen as a non-negotiable part of life, just like diet and sleep.**

By shifting perspectives and integrating **strength training into daily routines**, Indians can build healthier, stronger communities and enhance longevity.

LONG-TERM STRENGTH & WELLNESS STRATEGY

Aging is inevitable, but losing strength and vitality doesn't have to be. Developing a sustainable strength and wellness strategy ensures long-term fitness and health, helping individuals stay active and strong well into old age. This chapter covers the importance of consistency, tracking progress, and adopting a fitness mindset that lasts a lifetime.

Staying Consistent with Workouts as You Age

Consistency is the foundation of long-term fitness. As individuals grow older, their exercise routines must adapt to their changing needs, but the fundamental principle remains the same: **keep moving and stay strong.**

1. **Setting Realistic Goals**

> ➤ Define **achievable, long-term fitness goals** based on age, lifestyle, and health conditions.

➢ Shift focus from aesthetics to **functional strength, mobility, and overall well-being.**

2. **Prioritizing Strength Training in Every Life Stage**

   ➢ **20s-30s:** Focus on building muscle and strength, establishing lifelong habits.

   ➢ **40s-50s:** Maintain muscle mass, focus on injury prevention, and refine mobility.

   ➢ **60s & beyond:** Prioritize joint health, flexibility, and maintaining daily functional movements.

3. **Creating a Flexible Workout Routine**

   ➢ Workouts should be **adaptable** to changes in energy levels, injuries, or lifestyle shifts.

   ➢ **Weekly Plan:**

      o 3-4 days of strength training.

      o 2-3 days of mobility and flexibility work (yoga, Pilates, stretching).

      o Active recovery days (walking, swimming, or low-impact sports).

4. **Overcoming Barriers to Exercise**

   ➢ **Time Management:** Schedule workouts as non-negotiable appointments.

   ➢ **Motivation Slumps:** Have accountability partners, fitness apps, or group training sessions.

   ➢ **Health Setbacks:** Modify workouts instead of stopping altogether.

How to Track Progress and Make Adjustments

Tracking fitness progress ensures continual improvement and helps identify areas that need adjustments.

1. **Measuring Strength Gains**

   ➢ Track **weights lifted, repetitions performed, and endurance improvements.**

   ➢ Use apps or workout journals to monitor progression.

2. **Body Composition and Mobility Tests**

   ➢ Take **monthly progress photos** or measure waist and muscle circumference.

➢ Perform **mobility and flexibility tests** to ensure joints and muscles remain functional.

3. **Energy Levels and Recovery**

➢ **How do you feel after workouts?** Fatigue and slow recovery indicate the need for more rest or nutrition adjustments.

➢ Track **sleep quality, stress levels, and post-workout recovery times.**

4. **Making Necessary Adjustments**

➢ If progress slows, adjust training intensity, **try new exercises**, or change workout frequency.

➢ Modify **diet and supplementation** based on recovery and performance indicators.

➢ Incorporate **deload weeks** (lighter workouts every few months) to avoid overtraining.

Developing a Sustainable Fitness Mindset for Lifelong Health

Long-term wellness isn't just about exercise—it's about building a lifestyle that fosters physical and mental resilience.

1. **Shift from Short-Term Motivation to Long-Term Discipline**

   ➤ Understand that **fitness is a lifelong journey, not a short-term fix.**

   ➤ Find joy in movement—whether it's strength training, yoga, or outdoor activities.

2. **Prioritize Mental and Emotional Health**

   ➤ Strength training **boosts mood and reduces stress**, helping develop a positive mental outlook.

   ➤ Meditation, mindfulness, and recovery techniques enhance long-term fitness success.

3. **Making Fitness a Lifestyle Habit**

   ➤ **Incorporate movement into daily routines:** Walk instead of drive, use stairs, stretch during work breaks.

   ➤ Surround yourself with a **supportive fitness community** to stay inspired.

4. **Nutrition, Sleep, and Recovery as Pillars of Longevity**

   ➤ A **balanced diet** fuels the body for strength and endurance.

> ➤ **Prioritize sleep** to optimize muscle repair, hormone regulation, and mental clarity.

> ➤ Engage in **active recovery practices** such as stretching, massages, and hydration.

Final Takeaways: Building Strength for a Lifetime

> ➤ **Consistency in workouts** is key to maintaining strength as you age.

> ➤ **Track progress and adjust workouts** based on strength levels, recovery, and health needs.

> ➤ **A sustainable fitness mindset** ensures lifelong physical and mental well-being.

> ➤ **Prioritize movement, nutrition, and recovery** to optimize strength, prevent injury, and support longevity.

By embracing **strength training as a lifelong commitment**, individuals can maintain vitality, independence, and overall well-being well into their senior years.

CONCLUSION: THE PATH TO STRENGTH & LONGEVITY

Key Takeaways on Strength Training and Hormone Optimization

Strength training and hormonal balance are two of the most powerful tools for maintaining long-term health and vitality. Throughout this book, we have explored the science behind strength training and how it interacts with hormones to optimize physical and mental well-being. Here are the essential lessons:

- **Muscle Is a Key to Longevity:** Strength training preserves lean muscle mass, enhances mobility, and prevents age-related degeneration.

- **Hormones Are the Regulators of Health:** Testosterone, growth hormone, cortisol, and insulin play crucial roles in energy, metabolism, and muscle recovery.

- **Nutrition Supports Hormonal Health:** Protein-rich diets, micronutrients, and traditional Indian foods can enhance hormone balance and muscle recovery.

➤ **Recovery Is as Important as Training:** Sleep, stress management, and proper rest allow muscles to rebuild and hormones to stabilize.

➤ **Strength Training Benefits All Ages:** Whether in your 20s or 70s, resistance training can help improve quality of life and reduce the risk of chronic diseases.

By following a structured and sustainable strength training regimen, individuals can ensure long-term health and vitality.

The Importance of Patience and Long-Term Commitment

One of the biggest mistakes people make in fitness is expecting quick results. The path to strength and longevity is built over years, not weeks. Understanding the principles of **progressive overload, consistent training, and balanced nutrition** will help individuals stay committed for the long haul.

1. **Strength Gains Take Time**

➤ Expect small improvements each month rather than dramatic overnight results.

> Consistency is more important than intensity—stick to a program that is sustainable for life.

2. Avoiding Burnout and Injuries

> Overtraining can lead to injuries and setbacks. Listen to your body and rest when needed.

> Periodization (changing training phases) ensures continued progress without burnout.

3. Overcoming Setbacks

> Plateaus, minor injuries, and motivation dips are normal.

> Focus on **small wins**—increased endurance, improved form, or better recovery times.

A Practical Roadmap to Aging Strong and Staying Fit

Aging doesn't mean becoming weaker or less active. With the right approach, individuals can maintain—and even enhance—strength, mobility, and endurance as they grow older.

1. Strength Training for Different Life Stages

> **20s-30s:** Build a strong foundation with progressive overload training and muscle-building.

> **40s-50s:** Focus on maintaining strength, preventing injuries, and optimizing recovery.

> **60s and Beyond:** Prioritize joint health, flexibility, and functional fitness to maintain independence.

2. Daily Habits for Lifelong Strength

> **Move Every Day:** Whether it's a structured workout, yoga, or walking, staying active is key.

> **Prioritize Nutrition:** Eat whole foods, sufficient protein, and micronutrients for optimal hormone function.

> **Improve Sleep and Recovery:** Aim for **7-9 hours of sleep per night** and incorporate stress-relief activities.

3. Creating a Sustainable Routine

> Find workouts you enjoy, whether it's weightlifting, bodyweight exercises, or traditional Indian activities like wrestling or yoga.

> Incorporate **social fitness**—workout with family, join a gym, or participate in community wellness programs.

> Use **tracking tools** to monitor progress and adjust your approach as needed.

Final Thoughts: A Stronger, Healthier Future

Strength training and hormonal balance are **life-changing tools** for improving longevity and overall well-being. Aging does not mean losing vitality—it's an opportunity to continue building resilience and strength.

By focusing on **progress over perfection**, prioritizing **long-term consistency**, and making **strength training an integral part of daily life**, individuals can ensure a future filled with energy, health, and independence.

Start today. Stay consistent. Stay strong

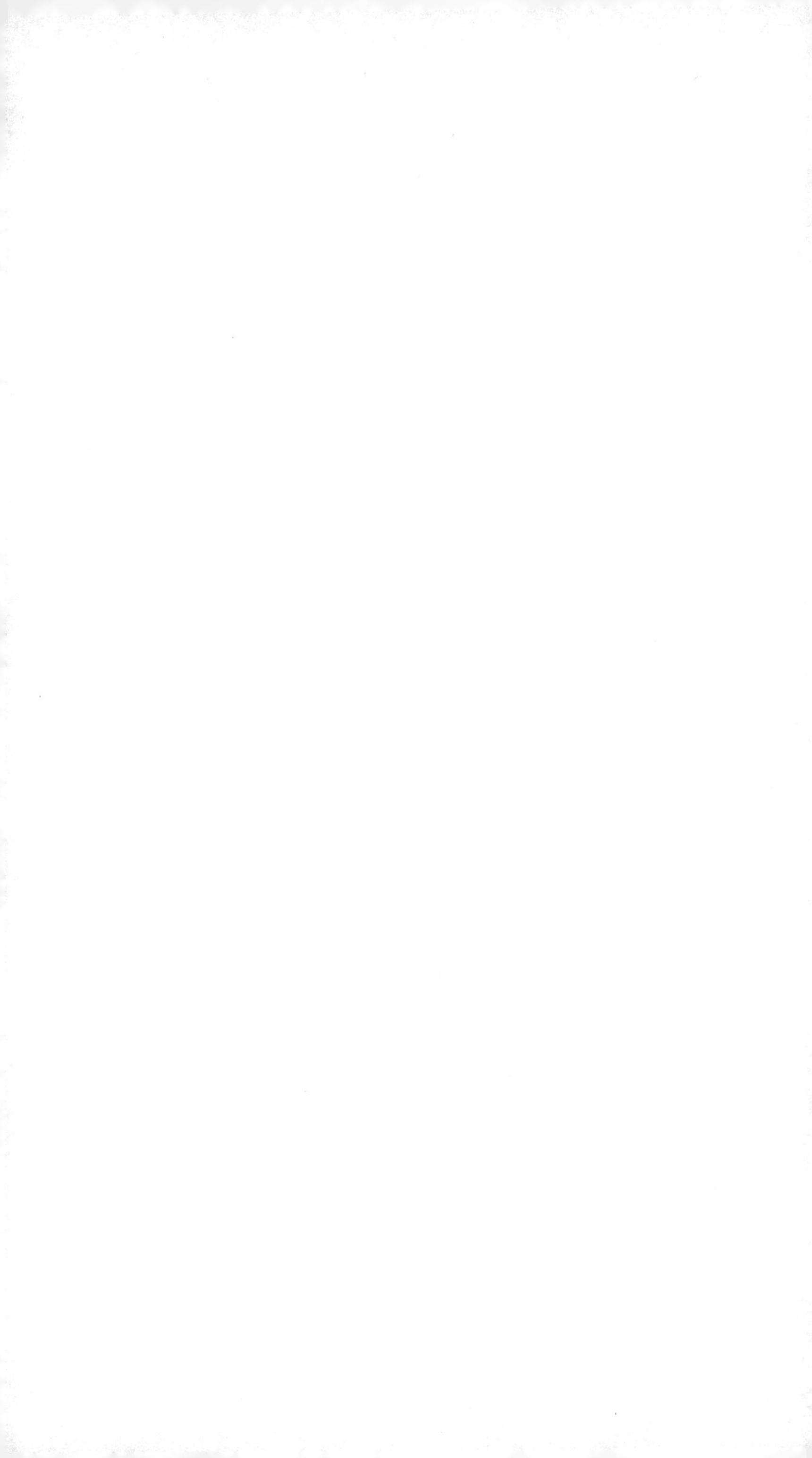